The Little Stress-Relief Workbook

The Little Workbooks series

The Little ACT Workbook

The Little Anxiety Workbook

The Little CBT Workbook

The Little Depression Workbook

The Little Mindfulness Workbook

The Little Self-Esteem Workbook

The Little Stress-Relief Workbook

The Little
Stress-Relief
Workbook

Jess Henley

crimson

Important note

The information in this book is not intended as a substitute for medical advice. Neither the author nor Crimson Publishing can accept any responsibility for any injuries, damages or losses suffered as a result of following the information herein.

The Little Stress-Relief Workbook

Published in 2020 by Crimson
An imprint of Hodder and Stoughton
An Hachette UK company

© Jess Henley, 2020

British Library Cataloguing in Publication Data

A catalogue record for this book is available from the British Library

Trade paperback ISBN 978 1 780592 85 5
ebook ISBN 978 1780592 86 2

Typeset in Whitney HTF by Hewer Text UK Ltd, Edinburgh
Printed and bound in Great Britain by Clays Ltd, Elcograf S.p.A.

Hodder & Stoughton policy is to use papers that are natural, renewable and recyclable products and made from wood grown in sustainable forests. The logging and manufacturing processes are expected to conform to the environmental regulations of the country of origin.

Hodder & Stoughton Ltd
Carmelite House
50 Victoria Embankment
London EC4Y 0DZ

www.hodder.co.uk

For all my clients who continuously teach and inspire me to work constantly on expanding my knowledge. And for my family who have supported me every step of the way.

Contents

About the author

Jess Henley has been working as a psychotherapist for the past 10 years and runs her own private practice in London. She completed her training and transpersonal psychotherapy masters at the Centre for Counselling and Psychotherapy Education (CCPE). Her thesis explored the transformative and healing power of humour. Her approach is integrative, combining the power and information of both the body and mind to help her clients unravel the jumble in their lives to find clarity, strength and peace. She believes that the key to learning is to be constantly curious and open-minded about the self and others, which can then enable healing and personal growth in any situation. She is a published journalist and writes a regular therapy column.

Introduction

Stress. Such a tiny word but it carries so much weight. Experienced by everyone in some capacity, it can both help and hinder your life. Stress is part and parcel of our modern-day existence but becoming unwell and being signed off work due to stress is more and more common. How can we identify stress and stop it in its tracks before it takes over? *The Little Stress-Relief Workbook* aims to help you understand how *you* uniquely respond to stress and teach you how to deal with it, so it doesn't need to have such a powerful impact on your life.

Fight, flight or freeze response

When we're feeling stressed, the brain sends signals for the body to release your stress hormones – the ones that trigger the fight or flight response. The fight or flight response is inherited from our ancestors and, when we sense danger, it signals to our body either to get ready to stay put and fight, or to get ready to flee to safety. Generated in our sympathetic nervous system when our adrenal glands are activated, it leads to increased heart rate, rapid breathing and increased blood pressure. A lesser-known reaction, but just as common, is to freeze instead of fight or flight. Your mind goes blank, and you literally feel like your whole body won't move or do what you want it to do, you've frozen in time. It comes from that animalistic response of 'playing dead', so any predators – or the stress trigger – won't spot you and will move away.

Stress is a valuable and critical response, it's reassuring to know that instinctively our minds and bodies will work together to help us get out of danger. However, our stress response cannot differentiate between what is real and what is imagined. Therefore, our bodies often go into this heightened state when it's not necessary, and if this continues over the long term then we start to suffer both physically and mentally as our minds and bodies never have the chance to get back into a state of equilibrium.

Different types of stress

Acute stress is short-term stress and occurs as a direct result of a specific event. It can come from anything unexpected, such as your train being cancelled, an argument with your partner, a near miss in a car or forgetting an appointment. This type of stress can be useful as it galvanises you into action, makes you think on your feet and motivates you to get things done.

Chronic stress is when your stress is ongoing and has built up over time. You've had repeated exposure to your stress trigger and you are living in a heightened state of stress arousal. It's this type of stress that can have long-term effects on your health, and it is chronic stress that we shall focus on in this book. This book will help you learn how to identify both your stress triggers and your responses to those triggers, and teach you how to manage those responses so you can bring yourself back to a non-stressed state.

Stress versus anxiety – what's the difference?

Chronic stress and anxiety are very closely linked, and many people aren't sure how to differentiate between the two. Both chronic stress and anxiety carry a lot of the same symptoms but the key difference is: stress has a trigger whereas anxiety doesn't. Anxiety is a feeling of fear, unease and worry and can latch itself onto anything in order to get felt. If you are suffering from stress not anxiety, then, regardless of whether it's acute or chronic stress, if you can relieve yourself from the trigger the stress response will drop away and you should start to feel better.

However, continuous stress (chronic stress), by virtue of its unrelenting nature, can lead to anxiety that doesn't then fade once the stress trigger has been overcome. Everyone experiences stress at different points in their lives, and often it can be chronic and ongoing, but if you start to notice it spilling out into other areas of your life beyond your response to the stress trigger, and it starts impinging negatively on your daily life, then you might be suffering from anxiety, and in that case I would encourage you to seek additional or alternative help.

How to use this book

The Little Stress-Relief Workbook is designed to give you a selection of practical tools to help you identify what your stress triggers are, then teach you how to work with them. The book works with both the body *and* the mind, so you can learn to understand how your whole being reacts to stress, not just how it affects your thoughts.

This book requires you to use your imagination in a way that could be unfamiliar to you. By tapping into your imagination you can learn to bypass the repetitive thoughts that don't bring you any solutions, and you can learn to work with your deeper subconscious to better understand your whole being.

If, at first, you struggle with any of the exercises or they seem a bit abstract to you, then I encourage you to put judgement aside, take a leap of faith and trust that your mind will take you where it wants to go and find the right mental images for you. There are no rights or wrongs in your imagination.

With each exercise, take your time reading each stage and allow the concepts and ideas to sink in and percolate through your mind before moving onto the next exercise. If it helps, record each exercise onto your phone so that you can have a running dialogue talking you through each stage instead of having to constantly refer back to the book.

Learning to breathe properly (Chapter 3) is central to this book and all the exercises within it, so take your time to really concentrate on how to do this, and don't move forwards until you feel you've got it nailed.

Some of the chapters will resonate more with you than others, that's normal. Once you've identified a few techniques that really work for you, then channel your energy here and keep practising. Once these become second nature, you can then go back to the other techniques. Also, once you've practised enough, you will notice that you can start combining the exercises. For example, living in the now (Chapter 4) will help you say goodbye to 'should' (Chapter 5), as well as give you more perspective on your core beliefs (Chapter 2).

Keep checking in with yourself

Most importantly, remember being stressed doesn't have to be a way of life. You may notice your stress starts to drop away little by little, and to start with you might not notice significant improvements. Help encourage yourself by spotting the small changes first; for example, it might be that you were stressed for only twenty minutes of a thirty-minute meeting, whereas before you would have been stressed the whole way through; or maybe your heart started pounding a little later than usual when you were confronted by a family scenario you usually try to avoid. Once you start to notice the little changes, these can empower you to realise that change *is* possible. And small changes can encourage you to keep persevering with the exercises in this book so you end up with the larger life changes that you're seeking.

Of course, there may be some scenarios where totally cutting your stress trigger out of your life rather than just managing it is what is required – it might be that you should quit your job, stop interacting with someone who triggers you, end a relationship – but I would encourage you to work through the exercises in this book first so that you can make any life-changing decisions from a place of deeper self-awareness, which in turn will help you feel more grounded, stable and confident in those decisions.

1 Identify your stress triggers

Stress manifests itself both mentally and physically, and how exactly it manifests is different for every one of us. In order to help reduce stress, you need to find out where it is in your body and how it's playing out for you. The key is realising your mind and body are one; they are not two separate entities as so many people believe. Once you can listen to your whole being, mind and body together, then you can start to make significant strides in helping reduce stress in the long term.

Tuning into your body

For so many of us our mind and body are disconnected from each other. The belief is often: 'It's mind over matter, I can think my way out of this, I'll push through this pain even though my body is screaming out to me to stop.' In actual fact, the optimum way to function is to have a mind–body connection – so that with your mind, you can listen to the whole host of information that your body is giving you all the time.

Have you ever noticed getting butterflies in your stomach before you've even realised you're nervous about anything? Or started blushing about something you thought you were okay with? Your body is telling you something even before your mind has made the connection. Your body is sending you these types of signals all the time and once you learn to listen to them, then you can learn to work with them.

And the best bit? Your body can't lie. It is telling you exactly how you *really* feel in that moment, when your mind might be telling you otherwise. Your mind can lie to you about all sorts of things: 'That person hates me', when they really don't; 'I'm really bad at my job', when you're actually very good at it; 'I'm never going to meet a partner', when you have no idea if that's true or not. If you can learn to tune into your body and start listening to what it's telling you, you'll have a much greater understanding of what's actually going on for you, and you'll be able to help yourself start to feel more grounded, calmer and less stressed.

How our bodies talk to us

When we are stressed our bodies can let us know in a number of different ways, but often we let our minds override this information if it is inconvenient. For example, your body is telling you need to rest but your mind is saying, 'No, I don't have time. I need to prep for this meeting, I need to leave work on time to pick up the kids, feed them and put them to bed. And then I need to work some more.' What happens next is that, instead of feeling better that you've managed to squeeze everything in, tiredness takes over (which is your body resending you the signal that you really need to rest). But, again, instead of listening to your body, you start to fuel it with caffeine and anything else that will help you stay awake. In response, your body, in a bid to get heard, shouts louder and sends you other messages it hopes you'll listen to; you start to get eczema breakouts on your skin, or your hair starts falling out, or you notice a part of your body that is slightly weaker starts to ache a lot more and starts causing you physical pain and increases your feelings of stress. Again, your body is using these physical signals to shout out to you to just STOP and REST. But you don't, you push on through. This can go on and on with physical ailments getting worse and worse as our bodies shout louder and louder in order to get heard.

If you can learn to tune into your body and pick up on the early signals and listen to them, then you can avoid everything escalating. Of course, you might not be able to rest in the exact moment that your body is telling you to, but you *can* acknowledge that resting is a priority, and that you need to slow down, give yourself a break and make sure you factor this into your weekly schedule wherever possible.

Robert (35) was feeling very stressed trying to juggle work, a newborn baby and buying his first house all at the same time. He noticed his skin was flaring up, he constantly had an upset stomach and he was always exhausted. Our therapy started with helping him tune into his body - as he talked through various issues, we would check in and see what he was feeling in his body. We discovered that when he was talking about work he always held his stress in his stomach - he noticed his stomach would tighten and that it felt like a ball of thorns was twisting and curling in there. He started using the techniques included in this book and learnt to bring his stress levels down. He noticed the ball of thorns gradually softened and his upset stomach slowly cleared up. Once he was able to see how his mind and body were connected, he started to use his body as a guide to tell him how he was feeling. When his skin started to flare up, he would check in with himself and try and identify the stress trigger so he could work to bring those stress levels down. He would then notice his skin would start to clear up again. Over time, as his stress levels reduced significantly, he was amazed to discover how much stronger he felt in his body overall.

Exercise 1.1
What are my physical stress responses?

The first step is learning to identify your own unique physical responses to stress. Once you start listening to your body you can start to spot what your stress triggers are.

- Imagine a scenario that you know makes you stressed – it might be flying, presenting in a meeting, social gatherings, etc.

- Close your eyes and, working in the present tense, imagine you are stuck right in the middle of your stressful scenario.

- Notice everything that happens to you physically when you're in that situation – you might be short of breath, sweating, stumbling over your words.

- Try and connect with the physical sensations that are happening to you in that moment and this will tell you a number of your physical responses to stress.

- Repeat the exercise with another, different scenario and notice if you have the same responses or if they differ slightly.

With this exercise you are beginning to bring awareness to your body, which is the first step of being able to tune in and listen to what your body is trying to tell you. The more you practise, the easier it'll become.

Typical physical stress responses

- Rapid heartbeat
- Sweating
- Rapid breathing
- Feeling hot
- Stomach ache
- Hair loss
- Skin scratching

- Eating junk food
- Drinking alcohol
- Smoking
- Headaches
- Migraines
- Insomnia

Noticing stress trigger patterns

Spend the next week or two tuning into your body and noticing each time you have a physical response to something and note it down. After a while you may start to notice patterns forming about when and under what circumstances your stress response gets triggered. You might notice that you always get hot and bothered before meeting a new group of people, or you may notice that you reach for the biscuit tin every time you have to ask for help. This tells you what your stress triggers are (new people, asking for help) – then, with this new awareness, you can start to work more deeply, with the techniques you'll learn in this book, on the issues that trigger you.

Exercise 1.2
What are my stress triggers?

Note down all the things that make your stress levels rise. Don't worry if these overlap or repeat themselves. It will be helpful for you to see patterns forming.

- ....
- ....
- ....
- ....
- ....
- ....

- ....
- ....
- ....
- ....
- ....
- ....
- ....
- ....

Are your triggers external or internal?

Once you've got your list of stressors, you can break them into two categories, those that are external – things from outside of you that are making you feel stressed – and those that are internal or evoked from within.

Examples of external stressors:

- *Work* – the number of emails you get every day, the boss you don't like, your commute, speaking in meetings, deadlines.

- *Environment* – loud noises, the weather, being among other stressed people, environmental disasters such as earthquakes, flooding, etc., the news.

- *Major life changes* – getting married or divorced, becoming a parent, being in an accident, your child being in an accident.

- *Socialising* – speaking to strangers, going on a date, other members of your family, work events.

Examples of internal stressors:

- *Beliefs, attitudes, perceptions* – thoughts and beliefs about yourself and others. Often when you're stressed these are distorted and exaggerated. For example, if you're stressed about meeting someone for the first time, afterwards you might only focus on the one 'stupid' comment you believe you made and totally disregard all the great things you said.

- *Fears and phobias* – concerns about what might happen to you or your loved ones in any given situation. Again, the scenarios are most likely distorted from reality, making them seem a lot worse than they actually might be.

- *Control* – feeling the need to manage a situation or the feeling of being out of control of a situation. Many people spend their lives trying to control things they can't, thus giving themselves a lot of undue stress. Superstitions are a great example of this – 'If I do X then Y won't happen'; this is just a way to feel as if you have control over something that in reality you have absolutely no control over. Instead, the superstition starts to have control over you, making you feel more stressed if you don't meet its demands.

- *Unrealistic expectations* – of yourself and others. When reality doesn't match up to an ideal in your mind then it can cause stress.

How to work with your stress

Knowing if your stress is external or internal is important as this can help you when you start to work with it. External stressors might have more practical solutions, such as limiting the amount of time you check your emails when you get home, or not allowing yourself to read the news after a certain time of day. Internal stressors are more complex, and they involve working to make your subconscious conscious so you can understand yourself better, which, in turn, will help reduce and relieve stress; the exercises in this book are designed to help you with that.

The key thing to remember as you work through each exercise, is to keep checking in with your body. Not only will it tell you how you are really feeling, but it can also be used as a map. For example, you may find that when you felt stressed about a regular event last month, you felt extremely nauseous, but this month, although you still feel slightly unwell, it may be minimal compared to before. This indicates that your stress response has reduced and you are coping better with the situation.

Projecting your stress onto other things

If it's not manifesting as physical ailments, stress can often be projected outwards on to something or someone else as a way to relieve it. You might notice yourself getting unreasonably angry at inanimate objects, or shouting at the dog or your child about something they don't really understand. If you notice that your reaction to something is disproportionate to what actually happened, then the chances are you're projecting something else on to that scenario. For example, you might notice yourself getting unreasonably frustrated with your child that they won't listen to you, but on reflection you realise you were angry and stressed at how your boss was ignoring you and wouldn't listen to you at work. There, you were unable to speak up, and so now you're reacting to your child in a much more dramatic way than the situation warrants – in effect, you are projecting the anger you feel at your boss on to your child as a way to get it out of your system.

Projecting your stress outwards can mean it infiltrates many more aspects of your life than it deserves to, and it can mean you feel stressed a lot of the time and not just when you are confronted by your stress trigger. Understanding the ways you project stress can help you notice it, reflect on it and calm down, allowing you to put boundaries down around the stress trigger and stop it from overflowing into the rest of your life. This will immediately help you feel less stressed as the stress won't be with you all the time, overwhelming everything. Understanding how you project stress will also make the real stress easier to manage as you'll know exactly where you need to work on it.

Johnny (44) had recently moved into a new place. He started to notice everything that was wrong with the house – the cracks on the walls, peeling paint, gaps above the skirting boards. This started to become an obsession every time he walked into his home. Were the problems getting worse? Had he made a huge mistake buying this house? He wasn't ever happy and content there, as all he could see was what might be wrong with it. After some therapy work, he realised he was stressed about all sorts of things in his personal life – his parents weren't well, his wife was struggling with depression, his job was being challenged. On the surface he seemed to be coping really well with all these other factors, but on reflection he realised he was projecting all the issues he was having in the rest of his life on to the house. Once he'd identified this projection, he was able to start working on the other stressors and his obsession with the house dropped away to a realistic level. Every time the house issues became exaggerated again, he knew it was a signal to himself that he was feeling stressed somewhere else in his life, so he would pause to reflect and identify the real cause and then start working on the trigger.

Ways you might project stress:

- Picking fights with your partner
- Beating yourself up about your physical appearance
- Feeling depressed
- Lack of motivation for anything
- Changes in sex drive
- Not wanting to socialise
- Becoming obsessive about something unrelated (as Johnny did with his house).

Exercise 1.3
How do I project stress?

Over the next two weeks, note down any ways you feel your stress levels are directly affecting your daily life.

- ....

- ....

- ....

- ....

- ....

- ....

- ....

- ....

- ....

- ....

- ....

- ....

- ....

- ....

Questions to ask yourself when you notice your stress symptoms flaring up

- Am I acting in proportion to what's actually happening, or could there be something else at play here?

- What's really going on for me right now?

- How am I feeling in my body when I think about this?

- What is my body telling me?

- What is really triggering me?

Once you've identified what the real trigger is, then, using the techniques in this book, you can work to bring down your stress levels and feel calmer and more grounded overall.

Summary

- Your mind and body are one, not two separate entities.

- Your body can't lie but your mind can.

- Your body can tell you when and what you're stressed about so listen to it!

- Identify your stress triggers.

- Notice when you are projecting your stress on to other things.

2 Core beliefs

The cause of stress is not only the external factors that are happening to you, but your perception of them; your *perception* of how you *think* you can cope with them rather than how you would actually cope with them. When you think you are being stretched to deal with something that you perceive is beyond your capabilities then your feelings of stress increase. If it's something that you perceive is manageable, then feelings of stress don't tend to manifest. Imagine you are being asked to present in a meeting. If it's on a topic that you are 100% confident about, then it probably won't make you feel stressed, but if it's on a topic that you feel you don't have enough knowledge on, then you might notice stress levels increasing significantly and a number of stress triggers might be activated – 'I don't know enough', 'I'm going to look stupid',

'Everyone is going to laugh at me', 'I won't be able to answer any questions after the presentation as I don't have the knowledge', etc. These stressful thoughts might not be accurate at all, but it's what you *believe* is true in that moment – it's how you are perceiving the situation rather than being based on anything factual. The good news is it's possible to change your beliefs – you probably have more knowledge than you think, you have time to access more information before the meeting, and no one thinks you're stupid or you wouldn't have been asked to present in the first place. The key is getting you to a place where you acknowledge the positive things, so they can help you reduce your feelings of stress and you can go into the meeting feeling calmer and more confident.

What are core beliefs?

When we are born, we are a blank slate. We don't have any beliefs about anything but as we grow up, we start to pick up beliefs from the world around us, primarily from our parents or primary caregivers; then, as we grow, from our peers, our teachers, society. These sets of beliefs govern how we function in the world on a daily basis. For example, if you were always told when you were little that spiders are scary or that carrots will help you see in the dark, then you will carry these beliefs with you unless you decide to challenge them at some point. Many beliefs are unconscious and therefore they drive our thoughts and behaviours without us really questioning them. Some of them are realistic – 'I believe I am capable of anything if I put my mind to it' – and some of them aren't – 'I believe I will fail at everything I put my mind to'. When we are stressed our negative core beliefs can take over and become exaggerated, making us feel like the challenge ahead is impossible; this then makes us feel more stressed and a vicious cycle of increasing stress and negative thinking ensues.

Examples of negative core beliefs

- I'm not good enough

- I'm not clever enough

- I'll never get that job

- I'm ugly

- I'm fat

- Things always go wrong

- The world is against me

- Nobody loves me

- I am unloveable
- I'll be single forever
- I must be perfect at all times

What are your core beliefs?

We all have thousands of core beliefs so it's impossible to name them all. Some will be deeply subconscious so you might not even know what they are, but the more you think about them and dig deeper to try to understand what belief is driving your behaviour, the more easily you'll be able to identify it and work with it.

How core beliefs can cause stress

Two people can find themselves in exactly the same scenario, yet for one person the scenario is stressful and for the other it isn't. This is down to how you *perceive* the scenario, rather than the facts of what is actually happening. For example, you're in the car with your partner on your way to a lunch party when you get stuck in really bad traffic which means you are going to be late. You are getting extremely stressed about the traffic and the idea of being late but your partner doesn't seem bothered at all, their mindset is there's nothing you can do about it so there's no point in getting wound up about it.

Some of the core beliefs that could be involved in the scenario and triggering stress for you are:

- being late means we don't care – therefore everyone will think badly of us when we arrive

- being late is disrespectful

- Mum thinks I'm lazy and being late will prove this to her

As you can see, how the situation is *perceived* by each you directly affects the level of stress you're feeling. Your partner doesn't have the same beliefs; your partner knows that being late is just unfortunate, as there was nothing you could do to control the traffic. Being seen as lazy or disrespectful as a result of being late isn't something that would ever occur to your partner as they don't have these core beliefs – therefore none of the same stress triggers are being activated and your partner remains calm and takes the whole situation in their stride.

Getting to your core beliefs

Since core beliefs are often unconscious, they drive our stress response without our knowledge. Once you shine a light on the belief that's triggering your stress, then you can consider it consciously and start to question it and see if it's really true. For example, using the situation above, if you consciously understand that the reason you're stressed is because you believe that being late is disrespectful, then you can start to unpick the whole scenario and disprove this belief which in turn will help reduce stress. You'll be able to see that you left an extra twenty minutes ahead of time so as not to be late, but there was no way of knowing that there was going to be an accident on the road meaning that the traffic would come to a standstill with no alternative route possible. As you had planned to easily be there on time, you are not disrespectful. Once you can follow this train of thought, then the stress that's related to this particular core belief should reduce as you have disproven the belief. You can take this method and try and work through each core belief one by one.

Exercise 2.1
Identifying my core beliefs

Think of a few recent scenarios that have made you feel stressed. Try and identify the belief behind the stress response and what feelings resulted as a consequence of being stressed.

Stressful scenario	Belief	Consequence (aside from feeling stressed)
Stuck in a traffic jam	I'll be late so I'm disrespectful. I'm lazy. I'm a magnet to bad luck.	Fear of mum's response. Anxiety about others' thoughts. Depression.
Presenting in a meeting	I don't know enough so I'm stupid. Others will laugh at me. I'll get found out as a fraud.	Embarrassment. Anxiety. Fear.

As you can see from the table, the stress response leads to a whole host of other emotions that are often linked to feeling stressed – fear, anxiety, depression, embarrassment, etc. So, if you can bring your stress levels down, then these other feelings should reduce as well.

Questioning your core beliefs

Now you've identified a few stress-inducing scenarios, you can start to question your beliefs with an aim of putting them in perspective.

- Separate out from the belief so it doesn't feel so personal to you. You can do this by imagining your best friend is coming to you for advice on the same issue. What would you say to them to help them see things more clearly?

- Pose the following questions regarding the belief.

  - What are the solid facts about the event? This requires listing only actual facts, and not ideas about what *might* happen or *has* happened. Using the traffic jam example, the facts are: I left twenty minutes earlier that needed, there was an accident, there was no alternative route, I have no control over the traffic.

- Are my stressful thoughts about the incident accurate? What evidence is there to support them?

- How could I think about this differently?

- How does it make me feel to think about this differently?

- When have I been in a similar scenario and how did that play out? E.g. 'No one even noticed I was late' or 'Everyone was sympathetic that I was stuck in traffic for so long.'

- When I've been in other stressful scenarios and everything has turned out okay, what internal resources have I relied on to get me through?

By answering all these questions, you should be able to identify how your core beliefs are affecting the way you perceive your situation and help you to realise how you could see things differently. There might be a number of core beliefs that are at play in any one given situation, so take each one on its own and work through each individually. Once you've done this with a few different scenarios, then you might start to notice that the same core beliefs keep rearing their ugly head – these ones might need more intensive work. As with all the exercises in this book, the more you practise, the easier it'll become. After a while you might start to notice that you identify familiar core beliefs a lot more quickly, so you can start working with them sooner and your stress response will hopefully not reach the same peaks that it used to.

Some core beliefs are so deeply ingrained in us it'll take a bit more work than just disproving them to reduce your feelings of stress. The other exercises in this book are designed to help you with that. For example, once you've identified a core belief and have disproved it, you can combine breathing (Chapter 3), living in the now (Chapter 4) and your safe place (Chapter 6), to help disprove your core belief on a deeper level.

TOP TIP

If you find it hard to think about how you might do things differently, then imagine someone who you do think would deal with the given scenario differently and better. Imagine exactly what they would do and what they would say, then channel that person so you can try and behave in the same way.

Summary

- Stress works on your *perception* of a scenario, not the *facts* of the scenario.

- It's our core beliefs that drive our perception of things.

- Making our core beliefs conscious is a way to work with them.

- Challenging our core beliefs can help change them and so reduce stress.

- If the core beliefs are deeply ingrained, combine this exercise with others in the book for a deeper, more transformative experience.

3 Breathing

Unless you've practised meditation, mindfulness or mindful types of exercise such as yoga and pilates, how you breathe might never have crossed your mind, but your breath hugely affects how you are in the world. We can survive for days without food, water or sleep, but we can't survive for more than a few minutes without our breath. Our breath feeds and nurtures all the cells in our body, carrying the correct amount of oxygen to where it is needed most.

Breathing is the essential foundation that you need for all the exercises in this book, and when we delve into ways to relieve your stress, we will refer back to this chapter again and again. If you can get your breathing right then from there you can build the tools to centre yourself and ease your stress levels. It's worth taking the time to practise perfecting your breathing so the rest of the exercises become much easier to do.

How our breathing is affected by stress

Our thoughts can influence how we breathe, and our breath then goes on to influence how our body functions. Ideally, we want our body to be in balance, but when we are stressed our body prepares for perceived 'danger' and goes into fight or flight response. As we've already discovered, this has an impact on us physically – our heart starts racing, we start sweating and our stomachs churn. Also, our breathing becomes short, shallow and rapid. This is to help us take in more oxygen so our muscles are prepped to flee, or to make us feel more alert and primed to fight. In most stressful scenarios in the modern world, fighting or fleeing is not what is required, so we stay in this heighted state of stress for prolonged periods of time. The oxygen then becomes unbalanced in our body, as it's not finding its way to the deepest part of our lungs, and this can lead to the physical symptoms of stress and anxiety. As you can see, it's a vicious cycle – the physical response to stress makes us breathe rapidly, which in turn perpetuates physical symptoms as the breath isn't going deep enough into the lungs to give the body the balance of oxygen it needs, and so feelings of stress can escalate.

What we actually need when we're stressed is to be able to take control of our bodies and calm down so we can function in an optimum way. This is where breathing properly comes in. If you can learn to breathe consciously and deeply then, when your body is in a stressed response state, you can learn to stop yourself going into full-blown fight or flight mode, and instead achieve a more grounded, calm state.

Exercise 3.1
Where do you breathe?

The first step to conscious breathing is to find out how you breathe in a non-stressful scenario.

- Find a place where you feel comfortable closing your eyes. Sit back, and with your eyes closed, focus all your attention on your breath. Notice everything about your breath: notice the temperature of the air as it passes through your nose; notice any scents or smells; notice the texture of the air – is it thick or thin?; notice how easy or difficult it feels to be breathing right now, in this moment, today.

■ Notice the speed of your breath – is it quick or slow? Notice where your breath is landing in your body – it might be high up in your chest, or it might be deep down in your abdomen. As you are doing this, if your attention wanders to other thoughts, then just label them as 'thoughts' or package them up in a balloon of any description, and let them float away – then bring all your attention back to your breath. It doesn't matter how many times your mind drifts, the key thing is to bring your attention back to your breath every time you notice your attention has wandered.

■ Now, consciously take your breath into your chest. Notice what it's like to be breathing in this place. Notice the physical effect it's having on your body – you may notice that you start to feel a bit lightheaded. Notice how long each breath lasts. Notice how nurtured the rest of your body feels. Also notice how natural it feels for you to be breathing into your chest.

■ Now, locate the place that is two inches below your belly button, and a third of the way into your body, consciously switch your breathing from your chest and breathe deeply into this place. If it helps, you can imagine there is a golden light that, with each inhalation, takes your breath through your nose, down the back of your throat and deep into your body. Notice your stomach expanding and contracting with each breath.

■ Make each breath last about eight seconds: four seconds to inhale and four seconds to exhale. Try and maintain this breath for as long as you can, and again notice how you feel in your body. Notice what's happened to any feelings of stress and notice any feelings of calm that might appear.

Which type of breathing felt more normal to you – chest or stomach? Which one was easier to maintain? This will tell you how *you* normally breathe, and everyone is different. If you naturally breathe into your chest then you are more likely to be susceptible to feelings of stress and anxiety as you are not feeding your body the optimum amount of oxygen it needs. By switching your breathing so that it's deep into your abdomen, you can instantly reduce symptoms of stress. Breathing into your abdomen can feel strange at first, but it's the most natural and best way for your body to breathe. When stressful feelings kick in, the body will start to fall into the abnormal pattern of breathing into your chest with short, shallow breaths.

Jo (33) came to see me as she was very stressed about going back to work after maternity leave. She found herself constantly worrying about how much her job would have evolved in her absence and how behind she would be. We practised the breathing exercise, and Jo realised she only ever breathed into her chest and she constantly felt on edge. At first, breathing into her abdomen was very difficult for Jo, and it took all of her conscious thought and effort. However, after a few weeks of practising every day, it became a lot easier; Jo noticed that although she was still nervous about going back to work, she also felt a lot more grounded and it felt a lot more manageable. She was amazed to see that by simply changing her breathing she was able to have a lot more control over her stress levels.

Practice is key

Breathing correctly has a cumulative effect so the more you practise deep breathing, the easier it'll become. Whatever you're doing, wherever you are – on the train, in a meeting, playing with the kids, going to sleep – you can practise your breathing. As soon as you remember to think about your breath, practise taking it as deep as possible. The more you do it, the more it'll gradually become second nature, and eventually breathing into your chest will feel like a strange way to breath. Over time, you should begin to notice that you get stressed less easily and when you do feel stressed, you will be able to use your breathing technique to help your body relax and the symptoms subside.

Exercise 3.2
Conscious breathing

Here is the technique again - you really cannot practise it too much!

■ Breathe deeply into the place that is two inches below your belly button and a third of the way into your body. If it helps, you might imagine a golden light that, with each inhalation, takes your breath through your nose, down the back of your throat and deep into your body. Notice your stomach expanding and contracting with each breath.

■ Make each breath last about eight seconds: four seconds to inhale and four seconds to exhale. Try and maintain this breath for as long as you can, and again notice how you feel in your body. Notice what's happened to any feelings of stress and notice any feelings of calm that might appear.

Rating your stress

Rating how stressed you're feeling can help put your feelings into context and make them more manageable. For example, compare how you feel physically and emotionally when you experience something that brings a lot of stress, such as nearly missing a flight, to something that should be low stress, such as being five minutes late meeting a friend. This can help put things in perspective and show that stress does not just function on one high-octane level. Then practise breathing into your abdomen for at least five minutes.

Exercise 3.3
Breathing when you are stressed

When you're feeling really stressed, rate your level of stress on a scale of 1 to 10 (with 10 being your most stressed). Then practise the breathing exercise above for at least five minutes.

Once you have brought your breath back into a deep, rhythmic state and allowed the effects to take place, once again rate how stressed you are feeling on a scale of 1 to 10. If the number has dropped at all, then you can feel empowered that you are taking control of your own stress response, it's not just something that is 'happening' to you. Once you can see evidence that the breathing technique is working, this can help motivate you to continue to practise breathing deeply whenever you can.

Quietening the thoughts

Of course, breathing can't take away the myriad thoughts swirling around in your head, but as your breathing becomes deeper and more regular, and as you focus all your attention on your breath rather than allowing your thoughts to take up all your attention, then you should notice that when the thoughts do appear again, they stop having so much power and therefore stop being so stress-inducing. Being able to empty your mind of thoughts and keep all your attention on your breath takes a lot of practice; even the best meditators in the world find their mind wanders, so don't be hard on yourself if you find it difficult to stay focused. Just be persistent, and every time you notice your thoughts intruding, consciously bring your attention back to your breath and what's happening physically in your body as you breathe. The more you practise, the easier it will become, and you'll begin to notice the time between your thoughts interrupting you gets longer and longer. You should also start to notice that a thought that would have led you to being really stressed before, just becomes more of a fact with much less emotion attached to it.

Using your breath in the moment

If you find yourself in a stressful environment, such as a family argument or an aggressive atmosphere at work, then you might need to take yourself out of the situation for a few minutes and regroup. Excuse yourself (go to the bathroom/take a phone call – whatever excuse you can think of to take you out of the situation), and find somewhere private where you can breathe deeply for a couple of minutes to ground yourself and regroup. If you're unable to remove yourself physically, then try to zone out of what's going on around you for a few minutes, or even seconds if that's all that's possible, and bring your attention to your breath and what's happening physically in your body. Slow your breath down and try and focus on counting your inhale and exhale (four seconds each), until you feel more calm and able to engage with the situation you're in.

Create a routine

Bringing mindful breathing into your daily routine can help reduce constant feelings of stress over time. Starting with just five minutes a day, try and build it into your morning routine. Perhaps before you leave your bedroom to start the day, set a five-minute timer and, sitting on your bed, practise emptying your mind and doing the deep breathing explained in Exercise 3.2. If you practise at the start of every day, you'll begin to notice that, over time, each day doesn't quite have the same levels of stress. You will also notice that when you are confronted with a stressful situation, you'll react to it in a more calm, balanced manner and the stressful feelings will abate more quickly.

Rex (46) found social situations extremely stressful. He would get very self-conscious when meeting new people and would sweat profusely, which would then increase his levels of stress and feelings of self-consciousness. As a result, he avoided socialising whenever he could. In the lead up to a wedding he had to attend, he diligently practised his breathing for ten minutes every morning for four weeks. He also practised breathing into his abdomen any time he remembered to during those four weeks. When the day of the wedding came round, he was still nervous about going and aware of the negative thought patterns that were circulating in his head;

however, he used his breathing whenever he started to feel overwhelmed, and he noticed that overall he felt a lot calmer, he sweated a lot less and therefore felt a lot less self-conscious. In turn, this increased his self-confidence, and he met and connected with a number of new people, something which he hadn't felt able to do in a long time.

Summary

- Breathing is the key to all exercises in this book.

- By helping reduce the physical symptoms of stress, breathing can help reduce stress levels.

- Breathing can help reduce the number and impact of swirling thoughts in your mind.

- Practise, practise, practise!!

- Create a routine so your breathing exercises become as natural as brushing your teeth.

- Simply changing your breathing can transform your life.

4 Live in the NOW

Stress (and anxiety) are usually based in the future or in the past – 'I've got to meet a deadline', 'I've got to clean the house/pick up the kids/do the shopping in the next hour', 'I had an argument and I don't know how it's going to get resolved', 'I've had a diagnosis and I don't know what's going to happen'. None of us know what's going to happen in the future, and we can't change the past – all we really know is what's happening right now, in this moment, today. For example, I know I'm sitting here typing this page, I know I'm feeling hungry, and I know that right now, in this moment, *I'm okay*. If I think about how much more of this book I have to write, how long that's going to take me and what my deadline is, then I can feel my heart rate increasing, my mind starts to buzz and goes a little fuzzy and I notice my stress levels increasing. But, if I stay with the fact that right now, in this moment, I am writing, words are going on the page and that I'm essentially okay, then being in the moment and living the reality of what's happening right now makes my stress levels decrease, my heart rate falls back to normal, I can think clearly again and I feel calm and grounded.

By living in the present, living from moment to moment, and by tackling things as they happen, as opposed to imagining how you're going to tackle them in the future *if* they happen, you can significantly reduce stress levels.

Stress in the future

Getting stressed about the future means not only do you have to deal with what will actually happen eventually, but you also put yourself through dealing with all sorts of scenarios that never *actually* happen, and so add a whole heap of unnecessary baggage to your mental load.

By cutting back to *only* focusing on what's happening in the present and only dealing with situations as they happen, you free up your mind of a whole lot of unnecessary stress.

Stress from the past

The same can be said about stress from your past. What's happened has happened. There's nothing you can do about it now. Sure, you can learn from your mistakes so you don't repeatedly fall into the same traps, but you can't change the past. Repeatedly reliving where you went wrong will only cause you increased stress.

The past isn't actually happening to you NOW – it's over. But if you keep on going over and over an unpleasant event from the past in your mind, then effectively you are bringing it into the 'now' – and why would anyone want to do that?!

By keeping your mind in the present, then you are able to leave all those stresses where they belong – behind you.

Johnny (43) had broken up with his wife three years ago, but he couldn't let go of what had happened and how he could have changed things. If only he'd said this. . . if only he'd done that. . . then maybe they would still be together.

The repetitive internal dialogue was causing Johnny to live in an active state of stress all the time. With his mind constantly in the past, he wasn't able to enjoy what was actually happening in his life and it was passing him by. By shifting his focus from the past into the present, he started enjoying life again. It started with the smaller things, such as the taste of a really good coffee in the morning, or the sound of the boy next door practising the piano. And the more Johnny practised being present, the more he noticed his enjoyment for the rest of his life increasing.

As this happened, and as Johnny focused less and less on the past, his stress levels reduced dramatically. He could still see how his relationship with his wife could have been different, but he was able to see it with some distance and perspective now as he was no longer living in a repetitive, stressful cycle of 'what if'.

Getting into the NOW

Some of us are never in the present, so let's look at what it feels like to be in the here and now.

Exercise 4.1

The object exercise

■ Find an object in your house and put it on a surface in front of you.

■ Set a timer for three minutes.

■ Focus all your attention on the object. Notice everything about it – the colour, how the colours change, the material it's made of, how it's fused together, how it sits, how it reflects light, what weight you imagine it'll be should you pick it up. Notice absolutely everything you can about the object's physical existence.

■ If any other thoughts intrude, once you've noticed them, let them go and bring your attention back to the object.

■ Once your three minutes is up check in with yourself. How are you feeling? How calm do you feel? How easy or difficult did you find the exercise? What was it like to be totally in the present?

- Once you find it easy to focus on an object for three minutes, extend your time to five minutes, then to seven minutes, and so on.

This is a very basic mindfulness exercise to get you used to living in the present, but you can take the theory and use it anytime and anywhere to help you get into the now, which will help reduce stress levels.

Noticing

When you're on your way to work start to notice everything around you. Notice the exact colour of the leaves on the trees, how the leaves are connected to the branches, how the branches are connected to the trunk, what colour the bark is, how you imagine the texture would feel if you were to touch it. Notice the buildings and every detail about them – the windows, the paint, the doors, how old/new/looked after they are. Notice the weather – how it feels on your skin. Notice what it's like to be wearing your clothes, how they feel on your body. Notice what happens to every muscle in your body when you move, when you sit on the bus or when you get squeezed between commuters on the train. When you get to work, notice what it's like to be sitting at your desk, what happens to your body when you're in that position, how your fingers feel as they work, what textures they are touching.

Whatever it is you're doing, bring your attention to every aspect of it as often as you can. This is truly being in the present and living in the NOW.

Be curious not judgemental

The key is to bring curiosity to everything, not judgement. For example, if you notice how your clothes feel on your skin, that's being in the present. However, if your mind then goes on to say 'They feel snug, therefore I'm really fat', that's adding extra dialogue based on one of your core beliefs about your *perception* of your body. Stay with the facts and your senses – the only fact you have in the here and now is how your clothes feel against your skin.

TOP TIP

As with all the exercises in this book, help yourself get into the present more quickly by using the breathing techniques you learnt in (Exercise 3.2, p45) – taking your breath deep into your abdomen and making each breath last eight seconds (four seconds to inhale, four seconds to exhale). Once you've connected to your body via your breath, then connecting to your other senses will have more impact.

Using the NOW to reduce stressful moments

Now that you know what it's like to feel present, you can start to apply this technique to any stress-inducing situation. If you're feeling stressed, anxious and nervous about giving a presentation, going on a date, taking a test, ground yourself by focusing all your attention on being in the present. Breathe deeply into your stomach and use a combination of your senses to get yourself off the merry-go-round of spinning thoughts about what *might* happen. Notice everything you can see, or the noises you can hear, or the things you can touch – whichever is the most appropriate sense for your situation.

If you notice your mind shifting and your stress levels increasing, then bring your attention back to what's actually happening in the here and now; keep coming back to the reality of the present. If you're taking a test and feel flummoxed by one of the questions, it can make your mind whirr into a spiral of disaster: 'I'm going to fail, then have to retake, but I don't have enough money to afford to do it again, so I'm never going to achieve my goal and I'll always be a failure'. Stop your mind in its tracks by bringing yourself right into the present. Notice the feel of the pencil in your hand, notice the feel of the paper in front of you, notice how the paper is fastened with a staple, notice how the paper sits on the desk in front of you, and keep your breath deep and even.

Once your mind has cleared and your stress levels have reduced to a more manageable state, relook at the question and see how it seems now. If it still seems impossible, then instead of letting your stress increase again, leave it and move on to the next one and be present with that one. By allowing your stress to take over, then all the rest of the questions can seem impossible; but by managing your stress and bringing it back down to a calm level, then even if one question remains difficult, the rest will be seen through a much clearer lens and therefore be easier to answer. Being present means taking everything just one step at a time, and slowly, slowly, almost anything becomes achievable.

Wendy (62) had a fear of travelling through busy cities and getting lost and stranded. Her daughter lived in London and was about to have a baby. The only way Wendy could get to her daughter's home was to take the Tube across London. The thought of doing this made Wendy so stressed that she hadn't been to London for ten years; but the draw of her new grandchild bought her to therapy to confront her fear. Wendy practised being in the present at home for about a month before her visit, starting with the object exercise. She then expanded being present to as much of her day as she could.

Wendy found that the stressful thoughts held less power if she stayed present. By the time she came to London, she was still anxious about her visit, but it felt manageable. She took every single aspect of the journey one step at a time – getting to the station, going down the escalator, checking out all the adverts, getting on and off the Tube and making two changes, until she made it to her daughter's station. She was absolutely amazed that she'd been able to do it and she said she felt invincible once she got there. At one point she'd got a bit lost but she'd focused on her breath, calmed down and asked for help with directions, which were happily given by another passenger.

By staying present and not allowing her thoughts to spiral into what *could* happen, to a future that would never even exist, Wendy kept her stress levels at a manageable level and achieved her goal.

Summary

■ Stress lives in the past and future NOT in the present.

■ Aim to be present in as much of your life as you can.

■ Use the object exercise to help you learn what being present feels like.

■ Expand the object exercise and be present in as much of your day as you can.

■ Being present will instantly help reduce stress levels.

■ Being in the NOW will give you perspective on stressful situations.

■ Practise, practise, practise! The more you can focus on the NOW, the more it'll become second nature.

5 Say goodbye to 'should'

How familiar is the word 'should' to you? Is it something you say to yourself a lot? Once you start to focus on it, many of us notice that we use it over and over, many times a day. 'I should be going to the gym', 'I really should start eating more healthily', 'I should lose weight, 'I should be more sociable', 'I should save more money', 'I should be more environmentally aware'. The list goes on and on. And what happens each time we 'should' ourselves? Well, we make ourselves feel stressed that we're not doing what we think we *should* be doing. If you were able to get rid of your 'should' dialogue, you'd instantly relieve yourself of a whole load of stress. Saying 'should' doesn't usually make you actually *do* any of the things it's telling you to. It just makes you feel bad about yourself that you're not doing them. There is nothing motivating about the word 'should'.

Negative 'should' mantras

Not just used in yoga, a mantra is simply a statement or a slogan that is used frequently. Due to the repetitive nature of a mantra, it can hold a lot of power, as you are telling yourself the same thing over and over again. Having negative mantras in your head about yourself induce stress, as you are telling yourself the same negative statement time and time again. 'Should' mantras tend to wear rose-tinted glasses: 'I should be more outgoing at work, then more people will like me and I'll be more likely to get a promotion'. None of this is factually true, people don't like you because you're outgoing but because of who you are as a person; also, you'll most likely get a promotion because you're good at your job, not because you're outgoing. If you can see the should mantra for what it is – a negative attack on yourself – and remove it from your mental dialogue, then you won't worry about how outgoing you are, and in turn you'll come across as more relaxed and confident, which will attract people anyway.

Jason (52) was extremely stressed at work as he was older than the majority of his colleagues, who were mostly in their thirties. He was worried that he wouldn't get included on the bigger projects as he didn't socialise that much through work. He tried going out with them in the evenings – as he felt he 'should' – but he never had a good time as he felt uncomfortable and out of place. We identified his 'should' mantras – 'I should be going out with the guys', 'I should be enjoying it', 'I should find them funny', 'I should want to be one of them'. In actual fact, he felt none of those things. Jason didn't want to go out with the guys, he wanted to go home to his partner; he didn't find them funny; and he certainly didn't enjoy being with them or want to be one of them. We started to unpick the should – whose voice could Jason hear in his head when he repeated one of the 'should' mantras? It turned out to be his father's. Over a few sessions he started to realise it was his father's expectations of who he should be at work that he was trying to live up to – rather than how he wanted to be. Once Jason was able to separate out from his father's voice and explore who he wanted to be in the office, he began to be more authentic; and once he started being himself, his confidence grew and he was much more relaxed. His colleagues all responded to this favourably, as they started to see him for who he really was and they liked and respected him for being different. Jason was also included on the bigger projects as, instead of being the same as everyone, he was now valued for the different perspective he could offer.

Stopping the 'should' dialogue helped Jason get in touch with who he really is, as opposed to who he *should* be; this reduced his stress levels significantly, and it helped him advance at work much more effectively as he was channelling the energy, which had previously been wasted on being stressed, into being more creative.

Exercise 5.1
What are your 'should' mantras?

Stopping your 'should' dialogue isn't easy. The first step is bringing *awareness* to it and how often you 'should' yourself. You need this awareness before you even start trying to change your habits.

- For at least a week, take note of every time you 'should' yourself and the circumstance around it.

- At the end of the week, have a look and see the number of times it happened.

- Notice when and under what circumstances your 'should' voice tends to have the most power.

- Notice what it's saying to you each time.

- Notice if there are any themes coming up among your 'should' statements.

- Notice how often it galvanises you into action or how many times it just makes you feel bad about yourself.

- Notice how stressed you feel each time you 'should' yourself but don't follow through with the action.

Each time you've used 'should' you're talking to yourself negatively. Would you talk to anyone else like this or criticise anyone else in the same way with the same frequency? If not, what makes it okay to talk yourself in such manner?

Cognitive distortions and how they create stress

A lot of stress is self-created by imagining what you 'should' be doing/thinking/saying as opposed to what is actually happening or possible. 'Should' statements negatively impact your self esteem; they are a cognitive distortion, as you never allow yourself the chance to see what you *have* achieved, focusing instead on what you think you *should* have. Cognitive distortions are the mind's way of disrupting our thinking so that we believe statements that aren't actually true. Most of the time, these distortions impact us in a negative way and lead to us feeling increased stress. For example, 'I didn't get that job as I mucked up the interview, I *should* have said X, Y and Z. I'll never get a job as I'm awful at interviews'. If you did genuinely perform badly in the interview, that does not mean you're awful at all interviews; it just means that in that moment, in that particular interview, you weren't able to deliver what they wanted. It does not mean that you'll go on to fail in every interview that you ever go to. However, the cognitive distortion tells you that it does, and this negative, polarised thinking could impact your performance in future interviews and lead to significantly increased feelings of stress.

'Shoulds' distort your thinking as they give you a list of rules about what *should* have happened, how you *should* have behaved, and what the outcome of any situation *should* have been. These rules bring with them feelings of stress and guilt when things turn out differently or when others think in different ways. More often than not, sitting on the sofa saying 'I should go for a run' isn't going to make you get your running gear on and head out of the door. It's just going to make you judge yourself negatively about the fact that you're not outside breaking a sweat. Take the fantasy away by removing the 'should' – 'should' statements are not factual. Once you remove the 'should' mantra and state what actually happened – 'I spent some time relaxing on the sofa' – see how you feel about the reality of the situation – is it really as bad as the 'should' part of you would lead you to believe?

Meet the 'should' voice in your head

Our thoughts run through our head as a dialogue, and every dialogue must have a voice attached to it in order for it to run. Often our thoughts have different voices attached to them according to the situation. For example, the voice you hear when you imagine how you are going to present your ideas in a meeting with your boss and your peers will sound very different to the voice you imagine when you think about putting your toddler to bed and reading her a story. When you tell yourself what you *should* be doing, with a bit of practice it's relatively easy to identify the voice that comes with the 'should', and often that voice can belong to someone you know – for example it might be your mum or dad's voice resonating from your childhood. Sometimes the voice doesn't attach to anyone in particular but you can imagine what that person would look like if they were a real person – for example it might belong to your typical stern matron-like figure who's cold and unrelenting, or the unrealistically 'perfect' idea of you that you have in your head.

Allan (38), had a particularly loud 'should' voice. After several therapy sessions, he was able to identify it as the voice of his father. Allan's father was a doctor, and had decided that medicine was the only path for Allan. Allan was an intelligent man, so working towards becoming a doctor was something he'd fallen into easily without much thought. When he started to come to see me he couldn't identify why he was feeling so stressed about his life.

On paper it looked picture-perfect. He owned his own flat, he had a loving long-term girlfriend, he was approaching the end of his training as a doctor and was applying for posts as a consultant. On working with his 'should' voice, Allan quickly realised that his whole life he'd been working towards what his father thought was right for him, what he felt he *should* be doing as opposed to what he actually *wanted* to be doing.

When he focused on a particularly emotive 'should' statement: 'I should be working at one of London's top hospitals by the time I'm forty', he realised that the 'should' aspect of that statement was coming from his father's voice, and hearing this voice made him feel like a young school boy, gagging for his father's approval.

Exercise 5.2
Change your inner dialogue

- Look back at your list of 'shoulds' from the week before.

- Notice what themes might have emerged – there may have been a lot around food/money/body image, etc.

- Starting with one particular theme, pick one of the 'shoulds' that feels the most powerful to you.

- Close your eyes, take a few deep breaths, focusing all your attention on your breath (as you learnt in Exercise 3.2), then hear yourself repeating the 'should' statement in your mind.

- Notice what the voice sounds like when you repeat the statement.

- If this voice goes with a person, imagine what that person looks like.

- Notice everything you can about that voice and the person it belongs to.

■ Notice how old you feel in yourself when you hear this person saying the 'should' statement to you.

Now that you've identified your inner dialogue and where it might stem from, you can start to change it.

■ Imagine yourself as a well-balanced, autonomous adult. If you find this tricky, then imagine a person you aspire to be who is calm, thoughtful and well-balanced. Imagine what their qualities are and embody them.

■ Once you can imagine yourself as this well-balanced person, have a conversation with the 'should' voice in your head.

■ Start by imagining the 'should' character and watch it repeating the 'should' statement to you. Then, from your well-balanced, adult position, respond by explaining to them why you didn't/ don't feel like doing what they think you should be doing.

■ Notice what the 'should' voice says in return and reassure it that you are capable of making your own decisions and that you don't need direction from the 'should' voice.

■ Ask the 'should' voice to step aside.

- Notice how you feel in yourself as the 'should' voice quietens. Notice what happens to your feelings of stress when you focus on what actually happened as opposed to what should have happened.

Allan's well-balanced adult took inspiration from a teacher he'd had at school. She'd been calm, friendly and very sure of herself and her beliefs. She was open-minded and willing to listen to others' opinions, but she always made up her own mind after much thought and consideration about how she personally felt about any given situation. Allan imagined himself embodying these qualities, then we imagined this new adult self having a conversation with his father. Over a number of sessions Allan tackled some of the smaller 'shoulds' – such as I *should* be dressed in a certain way – working towards the larger 'shoulds' – I *should* become a consultant. As his confidence grew in his new adult voice and he started to embody it more and more, he noticed his stress levels reducing significantly. Allan felt more in touch with himself and what he actually wanted from life. He realised that his passion still lay in the medical field but he wanted to work for a charity overseas, helping the most impoverished third-world societies, rather than in a private practice in a top London hospital. Once Allan had this realisation, although the journey to success would still be a tricky one with a lot of hard work, it didn't make him stressed as he felt truly connected to himself and what he wanted for his life.

Face the small 'should' mantras first

Just as Allan did, start by tackling the smaller 'shoulds'. The ones that don't have a significant impact on your life. For example: 'I should take the bins out tonight', 'I should clean up immediately after the kids have finished eating', 'I should iron the sheets even though it doesn't make any difference once I'm asleep'. Then once you're able to manage these ones and feel comfortable following what you really want rather that what you *should* be doing, start looking at the bigger 'shoulds', working your way up to the life-changing ones. For example: 'I should stay in this marriage for the kids', 'I should stay in this job as it pays well', 'I should go and visit my parents even though they're aggressive and rude to me'. Use the step-by-step approach to meeting the voice and opening a dialogue with it; if you still decide to follow what the 'should' voice says, then you are doing it out of choice, having consciously weighed up all the options, rather than because a subconscious part of you is driving you to.

Be kind to yourself

Quieting the 'should' voices is not easy, and just trying to block them out won't work. The more you block a voice, the louder it will shout. Remember, these voices may have been running your life for a really long time, so be gentle and compassionate with yourself. The key is to bring awareness to yourself and how often you are following the voices, not to judge yourself when you are driven by them. You might notice a voice saying 'You *shouldn't* do that. You're only doing it because the 'should' voice said so.' This is just another judgemental 'should' voice who needs the same treatment as all the rest.

Summary

- Your 'should' voice is a negative mantra.

- Negative mantras cause stress, not change.

- Identify your 'should' mantras.

- Meet the 'should' voices in your head.

- Learn how to respond to them from an adult, grounded position.

- Be patient, kind and compassionate with yourself through the process.

6 Find your safe place

Our internal world and imagination are very powerful places that can help us with a whole host of things, stress being one of them. Think about how often you daydream when you're feeling bored, or on the bus, or stuck in a traffic jam. This is our mind's way of taking us somewhere more stimulating than the reality of where we are – stuck on a train just outside our destination station for the fourth morning that week...

Harness your imagination

As well as taking us to luxury islands and giving us multimillion-pound bank accounts, our imagination can also take us to some difficult and unnecessary places as well – it can picture bad things happening to people we love, or activate phobias when there is no real threat. When we are feeling stressed, our imagination can go into overdrive. It can lead us to think about all the scenarios that might happen if something goes wrong. On the one hand this is the mind's way of being helpful, if you foresee every bad scenario and imagine how you can rectify it, then you're always prepared. But the reality is that every bad scenario isn't going to happen, so you're putting yourself through unnecessary stress. Your mind doesn't know the difference between you imagining the scenario and it actually happening, so each time you think the worst, which in a stressful scenario is often, your body is going through the same response as if you were actually in that situation. Take someone with a fear of flying, for example. When they experience turbulence, which is in reality no threat to their safety at all, their body and mind can still feel the same levels of stress, panic and terror as if they really were in an emergency situation.

If we can help prevent the imagination from jumping to the most stressful scenarios and take it to a safe place instead, then we can help reduce the stress response and feel calmer and more in control. Just as our imaginations can run away with us and evoke stress, so can we use our imaginations to harness peace and tranquillity. Rather than living a scenario that isn't actually happening, we can use the power of our imaginations to transport us to a stress-free safe place of calm that our bodies and minds will believe.

Tom (29) felt stressed around any kind of family gathering. He was the youngest of four and he hated any family meet-ups as he always felt belittled, picked on and never taken seriously by any of his family. He noticed that he would get very stressed in the days leading up to any gathering and this would manifest by him being very short, terse and cold with his girlfriend and co-workers. Usually a happy, outgoing man, he retreated into himself and became sarcastic and emotionless.

Through our therapy sessions Tom realised that this was his way of coping with his family – in preparation of seeing his relations he would step into a defended, hard persona a few days before. Through using a visualisation, we worked on finding Tom's safe place so he could use this imagery instead of having to retreat into himself. Once we established his safe place – which was his best friend's garden when he was ten –

he was able to use this image as a meditation for the few days before going to see his family.

By addressing the issue and working to take himself to a positive, safe place in his imagination, Tom found that he wasn't acting out towards those he cared about in the days before he went to his family. If he did find himself needing to mentally retreat from the world for while, instead of going into his cold, heartless place of old, he would consciously retreat into his safe place.

Tom was also able to imagine being in his safe place whenever he felt triggered by his family once he was with them. This had a huge impact: although he still couldn't find enjoyment in his family gatherings, the safe place made them a lot more manageable. Tom still got the same treatment from his siblings and parents, but now he felt protected from it, so it didn't affect him nearly so much. It also meant he didn't carry the negative feelings away with him when he left, so once he was back home, he was much better at shaking off the whole experience and stepping back into his life as a happy, kind-hearted man.

Exercise 6.1
Finding your safe place

Do this exercise at home in a quiet, uninterrupted place so you can really focus, then it'll be much easier to activate once you get into a stressful, triggering situation.

■ As before, focus all your attention on your breath, clear your mind and breathe deeply into your abdomen (See Exercise 3.2, p.41).

■ Imagine a place where you feel totally safe and at peace. Use whatever the first image is that comes to mind. Trust that your imagination will take you where you need to go, don't try and change it.

■ Notice absolutely everything about this place – tap into each of your senses – what can you see, what can you hear, what can you feel on your skin, what can you smell, what can you taste?

■ Notice what the weather's like, what the light is like, what time of day it might be.

- Notice if there is anyone else in there with you. If there is, it could be an animal, a person, a character from a movie or a book, an archetype.

- Notice how you feel in your body when you're in this safe space. Notice how peaceful and carefree you feel here.

- Breathe into the feeling of safety and see if you can locate it in your body. You might get a warm sensation in your chest/head/abdomen. Notice what it feels like to have this safety within you. It might feel like a warm glow, or like an area that is full of light. Whatever and wherever it is, breathe into this place and enhance these physical feelings as much as you can; allow them to flood the whole of your body and feel your being radiating safety.

Channelling your safe place

Now that you've got your safe space, you can use this imagery and access the feeling in your body whenever you are in a stressful situation that triggers you.

If it's a scenario that's planned, such as a meeting at work or going to the doctor or getting results for something, you can prepare yourself by doing a short five-minute meditation, imagining being in your safe place, every day for a week before the said scenario and then use the image just before you confront your stressful situation.

If you find yourself in an unexpected stressful situation, such as being stuck in a lift and you suffer from claustrophobia, then in that moment you can breathe deeply and bring up the image of your safe place and imagine that you are there and safety is radiating out of you.

Keep your breath deep and steady and notice how your heart rate is slowing – the feelings of stress should quickly become more manageable. As with all the visualisations, the more you practise visiting your safe place, the easier it'll become when you need it.

Bounce away negativity

Another time when stress can significantly increase is when you have to be around someone you really don't like or someone who has hurt you a lot in the past. It may be a work colleague that you just can't stand, or attending a social gathering where a former partner will be. In these cases, you might not be able to avoid seeing the person that triggers you, but you can use the power of your imagination to help yourself better cope with the situation. An imaginary protective armour will bounce off all the negative energy that you don't want to absorb from the other person.

Sarah (32) came to see me as she was being bullied at work by her boss. She held a director-level position and had a team of four people working under her. She noticed that whenever she was out of the office, her boss would make huge demands on her team that were not part of their jobs. When Sarah confronted her boss on this, her boss began a personal vendetta against Sarah and tried to make her life in the office as uncomfortable as possible.

Sarah was a very grounded individual who had done a lot of previous 'self' work and she could see that her boss's issue was not really about Sarah herself, but that she had become the scapegoat. Even with this understanding of the situation, life became very hard at work, as even though she knew it wasn't ultimately about her, the constant reassurance she had to practise with herself took a lot of energy.

We did a visualisation to help her find her protective armour and once we'd established this for her, she imagined herself dressing up in it every morning before work. Her armour was made of mirrors: she could imagine any negativity coming at her reflecting straight off her and back to her boss. It made her feel lighter and safer. Over time she noticed that her boss eased up on her. Her boss realised that scapegoating Sarah wasn't having the desired effect anymore and so she turned her attention elsewhere. Sarah was able to relax more at work and started to enjoy being there again.

Exercise 6.2
Finding your mirror armour

Do this exercise at home in a quiet, uninterrupted place so you can really focus, then it'll be much easier to activate once you get into a stressful, triggering situation.

- As before focus all your attention on your breath, clear your mind and breathe deeply into your energy abdomen (see Exercise 3.2).

- Now imagine yourself dressed in a suit of armour that is made up of lots of mirrors reflecting outwards to the world.

- Imagine every tiny aspect of the amour – how big each mirror is, how it moves when you move, how heavy it is, what colour it is, how it secures over your face, how it covers your back, what footwear goes with it.

- Notice how you feel inside it: how you move when you've got it on, how safe and protected you feel when you're wearing it.

- Imagine that you're wearing it in front of someone who is sending negative energy your way and notice the mirrors reflecting that negative energy away from you; notice that the negative energy is unable to penetrate you anymore and just bounces right off.

- Notice how it makes you feel to be protected in such a way; notice what happens to your posture when you're not being cowed by someone else's negative energy; notice how powerful and safe you feel when you're wearing your protective armour; notice how your stress levels reduce.

Practise at home

You can use this exercise, not only when you are directly experiencing someone's stressful energy, but also when you are imagining it. When you're at home and you feel yourself getting stressed just thinking about a scenario where you have to be in contact with your trigger person, imagine yourself mirroring off their negative energy. In your mind you can surround your house with mirrors too if necessary, to help stop yourself bringing all the negative energy home with you. This will allow you to leave the negative energy at the door, rather than allowing it to consume your thoughts all evening and impact you long after you've left the stressful situation.

Summary

- Your imagination can help reduce stress levels.

- Use your imagination to find your safe place.

- Learn how to locate this safety in your body.

- Use your imaginary safe place when you're confronted with a stressful situation.

- Find your mirror suit and bounce away negative energy.

- Practise at home so it becomes second nature.

7

Meeting your 'parts'

This is the most abstract of the chapters and will require the most thought and imagination, so take it slowly. If you find some of the ideas hard to get to grips with: pause, let them sink in, and see how you feel about them before moving forwards. Again, as with all the exercises, the more you practise, the easier they become; so try to persevere with these concepts as, once mastered, they have huge potential in being able to help you significantly reduce stress.

Which 'part' of you is talking?

We've all had those moments when, at the end of a long day, you get home and are just about to decide what to do for the evening and the phone rings. It's your friend inviting you to join them for a drink and a bite to eat. There's a 'part' of you that is so shattered all it can think of is bedding down in front of the TV, yet at exactly the same time, there's another 'part' of you that's saying, 'Come on, it would be fun to go out, let off some steam and be surrounded by friends'. These are two different aspects of your personality (or more technically, two of your sub-personalities) speaking up at exactly the same time. Our overall personalities are made up of hundreds of different sub-personalities – or 'parts', as we'll refer to them in this chapter – that work together to create the personality that we project to the world.

Our 'parts' are what makes us such complex human beings. We don't just think and feel in one definitive way with one resounding outcome: it's not either this or that, black or white. No, as human beings we're constantly evolving shades of grey. Our different parts can have conflicting emotions, desires, wants and needs all at the same time. For example, it's possible to feel both happy and sad simultaneously: happy that you're going travelling, but sad that you won't see your family for six months; happy that you've got a new job, but sad that you have to leave your old colleagues behind. And it's these conflicting 'parts' that make life so labyrinthine, surprising, interesting, but often confusing and stressful too.

How the parts work within us

All our different parts form a family within us, our internal family and, just as with any family, in order for it to function in a healthy way everyone needs to get their chance to speak up and to feel valued. Also, just as in most families, there will be some people (or parts of us) who have more prominence depending on the circumstances and what you're doing, and others who seem to sit more in the background. For example, the loud, boisterous part of you might come out every time you're in social situations, so many people would be surprised to know you also have a shy part that comes out when confronted with intimate one-to-one encounters.

When you're feeling stressed, it is unlikely that *all* of you is feeling stressed, there's just a part of you that is, and this stressed part has the most air-time at that point. If you break down how you're feeling into as many bits (or parts) as you can (and we're going to learn how to do that next), you might find that as well as the part of you that is feeling stressed, there are also a few other parts that have different feelings about your situation – a part of you that is proud of what you're doing, a part of you that loves rising to the challenge, a part of you that is daring and thinks 'feel the fear and do it anyway'.

By understanding all the different parts that are at play in any given situation, you can be empowered in the knowledge that although you feel stressed, you also have lots of other strengths (or parts) that you can call on to help get you through.

Julie (34) was very stressed about heading into a meeting with her male boss and two male colleagues who were her peers. She didn't understand why she was so stressed as she was confident with the material she had to present.

On breaking down the different parts of her that were being activated by the meeting, she realised that the part of her that felt stressed was the part that didn't want to be in the room with three men. She had been badly bullied in college by a group of men and found being without female company very stressful and uncomfortable.

On further investigation, she realised she had other parts of her that could help her in the meeting – the part of her that knew she was good at her job, the part of her that was an adult and could stand up to bullies, and the part of her that was extremely determined to prove herself at work.

Once she knew these other parts would be in the meeting too, she felt empowered, calmer and more confident. During the meeting she kept her breathing deep and steady, especially if she ever felt the stressed part being activated. By the end of the meeting she was delighted to hear resounding praise and respect from all three men in the meeting. And a stressful experience turned into a truly transformative one.

Exercise 7.1

Meeting some of your parts

The concept of having different parts to the self can be hard for some people to get their heads around, and this exercise can seem difficult if this whole concept is new to you, so try to be as open minded as possible. If you notice a voice saying this is all a bit far-fetched, then allow that voice to be heard, ask it to step aside, then try again.

- Sit back, relax and close your eyes.

- Following the same routine as Exercise 3.2, focus all your attention on your breath and allow any thoughts to drift away so that all your focus is on your physical being.

- Once you're feeling calm and present, imagine a scenario where you feel uncomfortable – it might be a meeting at work, a social gathering, a family meet up.

- Working in the present, imagine yourself walking into that scenario and notice how you feel – you might feel small, shy, self-conscious.

- Notice how old you feel when you're there. This could be any age: it might make you feel like a small child, a frustrated teenager or an exhausted grandparent (even if you're only in your thirties).

- Notice how you feel in yourself when you're there – you might feel like you want to hide or run out the room, or you might feel angry that you have to be there and you want to throw something.

- Notice what you're wearing when you picture yourself in this scenario and how you feel about your body: how comfortable do you feel in your own skin?

■ Keep breathing and notice everything you can about yourself in this scenario.

In this exercise you have met a part of yourself, this is one part of you that is showing up when you find yourself in this uncomfortable scenario. Now let's see if there are any other parts of you there as well.

■ Close your eyes again and take yourself right back to where you were in the scenario.

■ Ask yourself 'Are there any other parts of myself here?' See who steps in. You might notice a determined part of yourself who says, 'Come on, you can cope with this'. Or there may be a judgemental part that is whispering 'Don't be such a wimp'. Or an angry part might appear and encourage you to criticise everyone else in order to make you feel better.

■ Again, closely study each of these parts and notice everything you can about them – what they're wearing, how they're standing, how old they are.

This exercise helps you meet just a few of your parts – the ones that may be activated when you enter a scenario in which you don't feel comfortable. Now you can imagine any scenario at all and notice which of your parts are showing up. When you're running your daily life you can begin to notice which parts of yourself are in control during what times, for example, which part of you is activated when you get out of bed in the morning? It might be the parental part that needs to look after the kids, the career-oriented part that wants to get to work, or the resentful part that just wishes you could be in bed all day – or it could be all of these parts.

Spend a week trying to notice as many different parts as possible as you go through your day. Once you begin to notice them and the roles they play in helping or hindering you run your life, then you can start communicating with them, finding out what their needs are and how you can help them feel heard and valued.

Understanding your different parts

Many of our parts have different feelings and different motivations, but they have one shared goal: to do what they think is right for you. Think about the example of Julie (p.92). There was a part of her that was stressed to be in the meeting; this part was trying to warn Julie (through activating her stress response) that being around men could be bad; it was trying to save her from having a repeat of her experience at college. The confident part of her was helping by reassuring her she knew what she was presenting and she could DO this. Her adult part was letting her know that she was a grown woman who could stand up for herself and not be bullied. Her determined part was telling her – no matter what the men said – she could get through this just as she'd got through tricky situations before.

The most important thing to remember is that all of your parts have positive intent and want what they think is best for you, even if they come into conflict with each other, which can often happen. Just as in a normal family, one person (or part) might have one idea about what's best for you, while another person (or part) has a totally different idea. When this happens, you will notice that you find it hard to make decisions and you can end up feeling confused and stressed about your actions and plans. For example, if you have double-booked yourself to visit your grandmother at the same time as going to a festival with friends, a part of you might tell you that you should be going to your grandmother as she's getting old and needs the company, but another part of you says you should go to the festival as you've been working so hard you need some downtime and to let off some steam. In these scenarios, if you can learn to communicate with the different parts, you'll more easily be able to come to a decision you feel comfortable with, and this will help reduce stress levels.

Communicating with your parts

Many of our parts came into action when we needed them in order to survive, therefore they believe that what they are doing is for our benefit, even if this behaviour has now become destructive. For example, if there's a part of you that loves to drink alcohol, the positive intent could be that it helps to make you feel better by allowing you to avoid difficult feelings. The intent is positive but the outcome is destructive if you end up drinking too much too often.

Bearing this in mind, every time you communicate with a part of yourself the aim is to discover what that part's purpose is and to try to understand how it feels that it is helping you. Our aim is never to admonish or to cut off a part of ourselves; if you try to exile a part of yourself it will just come back stronger and louder. Our aim is to meet the part, listen to it and try to help it so that it doesn't feel the need to engage in destructive behaviours anymore.

Exercise 7.2
Communicating with your parts

- Identify a part that you want to communicate with. For example, the part of you that really doesn't want to go to work today.

- Sit back, relax and close your eyes.

- Following the same routine as Exercise 3.2, focus all your attention on your breath and allow any thoughts to drift away so all your focus is on your physical being.

- Once you feel you are connected to your body, ask if the part of yourself that you are working with minds stepping forward and going into a room on its own. This might seem hard to imagine doing, but once you're in a calm, meditative state your parts will usually show themselves if they want to. If you can't picture any physical being, then see if there is a shape, colour or sound that wants to appear. Once you're able to separate it out and can imagine it, then you can start to work with it. If nothing appears at all, the chances are you are trying to work with a difficult part, so open your eyes and start again with a part of you that is more obvious – such as the part of you that loves travelling, or the part of you that loves cooking – so that you can experience what it's like to talk to a part. Then, when you're feeling more confident, you can try to envisage the difficult part again.

■ Once your part is in the room, take in every detail about it – what it's wearing, how old it is, how big it is, what its posture is like, what emotion it seems to be carrying. If it's something more abstract, again use the same concept and imagine every detail of it that you can.

■ Next, give your part the opportunity to speak to you. Invite your part to say anything it wants by saying 'You can tell me anything. I am here to listen and not to judge, what would you like to say to me?' Don't over think this part of the exercise, just let whatever bubbles up come out.

■ Once you've started your dialogue, you can go on to enquire 'What's your purpose in my life?'; 'How do you feel you are helping me?' Remember to always thank the part for the work that it's doing. It will feel that its role is helping you, even if the behaviour has become destructive. Reprimanding your part won't be constructive.

- Keep the dialogue going for as long as you need to get as much information about the part as you can.

- Once you know how and why the part is acting in the way that it is, you can devise ways to help relieve it of some of the load that it is carrying; then it won't feel the need to act out in such a way anymore and you might notice your unwanted behaviours start to gently subside.

Robin (37) was stressed about leaving her one-year-old child at nursery for the first time. She knew it had to be done as she was going back to work and ultimately her daughter would be fine, but she couldn't let go of her intense feelings of stress. We asked her stressed part to step into a room on its own and it appeared as a young seven-year-old who felt helpless and vulnerable.

After opening a dialogue with this part, Robin discovered her anxiety related back to her own experience of being sent to boarding school at the age of seven, and her extreme feelings of abandonment. She realised she was terrified of her daughter feeling the same way as she had.

Now that she had identified this part of herself, she was able to reassure it that this scenario was totally different, that she wasn't abandoning her daughter and these feelings were from her past not her daughter's present.

Once Robin was able to put things into perspective using this technique, although she was still triggered by leaving her daughter at nursery, the feelings were a lot less intense and she was able to understand that the feelings were about her own story, not her daughter's, which helped reduce her stress to a much more manageable level.

How old is your part?

Noticing the age of your part is critical to how you communicate with it. If your part is six years old, you will talk to it very differently than if it were twenty-five or forty years old; always communicate with your part in an age-appropriate way. The age of the part will also give you an idea of how old you were when the part came into being and what was happening in your life at that time and why the part felt like it needed to step in to help you.

For example, if a fourteen-year-old discovered that the only way to be accepted at school was by playing the comedian, then the comic part will come into being to help that child survive in its surroundings. As an adult, being a comedian might then be a way to hide from all sorts of difficult feelings that were suppressed from the age of fourteen in order to be accepted at school – such as being shy or lonely. However, as an adult, these suppressed emotions might come out in a destructive way – such as depression and anxiety – which might seem strange to associate with someone who is known for being loud and funny. By communicating with the comic part, we can understand why it came into being, then we can reassure it that now, as an adult, we want to try and deal with the suppressed emotions. We can ask if the part would mind not disappearing, but stepping back so we can talk to the lonely and shy parts that it's protecting. This way the comic can still be a part of us, but it doesn't need to act as a guard anymore; and once the shy and lonely parts are properly accepted and dealt with, they can be healed and depression and anxiety can lift.

As you can see, we haven't tried to get rid of any part of ourselves, we have just relieved the parts from carrying their burdens. The resultant freed-up energy can be channelled into other more rewarding behaviours. However, it can be hard to unroot the reasons behind our different parts. If you're unable to get to them, don't be hard on yourself. The first and most important step is acknowledging their existence. If you don't succeed at communicating with a part you can always go back and try another time. Just as with any person, a part might not feel like talking all the time, so try not to give up. Just take a step back, regroup and try again another time.

Exercise 7.3
Working with your stressed part

Using the steps from Exercise 7.2, separate out the parts of yourself that get stressed. There may be a number of them: for example, there may be a part of you that gets stressed at work, but a different part that gets stressed when the kids are misbehaving, and yet another different part that gets stressed if you're unable to fall asleep. Each of these parts needs to be worked with individually. Once you've separated out the stressed part that you want to work with and put it in a room on its own, then you can start your dialogue.

Key questions to ask:

- What is your role in my life?

- How do you feel you are helping me?

- If I could ask another part to step in and help you, what part would you like to come along? (See below for some examples.)

Part of you	What do you look like	How are you helping me?	What other parts could help you feel less stressed?
E.g. Stressed part that needs to present in a meeting	Corporate	Keeping me organised	Adult part to reassure me
	Wearing a suit	Making sure I remember everything so I don't make a fool out of yourself	Confident part who knows what they're doing
	Hair scraped back	Keeping me on high alert so I don't get complacent and mess up like I did at school	Fearless part that doesn't mind making mistakes

Recruit other parts to help

The stressed part of you might have an idea of who can help it. For example, the part that is really stressed at work might say: 'If I was more organised then I could calm down a bit'. In this case, see if you can ask the organised part of yourself to step forwards. It might be a shock to you to find that you even have an organised part, as you may feel you are disorganised in every aspect of your life; but this could be because the stressed part has taken such a leading role that the organised part hasn't had the opportunity to show itself.

By using this technique, you are giving more parts of yourself a voice. You are giving them the space and freedom to step forwards, allowing them to help and take a more prominent position. Once the parts of you that can help have stepped forward, open a dialogue between the stressed part and the new part. Imagine them having a conversation and telling each other how they can work together and see if they can come up with a game plan of how to tackle the stressful situation. This might seem quite abstract, but it's just the same as imagining your parents or two friends having a conversation about something you know they have particular feelings about; you can literally picture how the conversation goes. Then, once you've established a new game plan between your two parts, you can put it into action.

Examples of parts you can recruit to help your stressed part

- Your *compassionate* part to help soothe your buzzing mind.

- Your *logical* part who knows being stressed won't get you anywhere.

- Your *determined* part for whom no job is too small.

- Your *grounded* part who can help you breathe properly and calm your body down.

- Your *wise* part who can put everything into perspective.

- The part of you that is able *to ask for help* when needed.

- Your *humorous* part who can see the funny side to everything and help you feel more relaxed.

In the moment

The next time you notice your stressed part being triggered, take a few minutes and focus all your attention on your breath, making sure you're breathing deeply into your abdomen as described in Exercise 3.2 (p.45). If you're able to go to a quiet space then do so, if not, then just notice and monitor your breathing wherever you are.

Next, bring to mind the part of yourself that is stressed, this should be quite easy now that you've met it before, as once you've made your parts conscious they will step forwards much more willingly. Ask this part what's going on for it in that exact moment. This part should then be able to tell you why it's stressed and what will help in that moment. Listen to the part, soothe it and reassure it that you now have a team of other parts that can help, and imagine them stepping in and working together. Keep up your deep breathing throughout.

If the helpful parts that you are recruiting are unfamiliar (such as the organised part in the example above) then be patient with them and give them the opportunity to do what they've promised to do to help. You might notice that the stressed part keeps screaming back at them – 'Hurry up, you're not helping, I still feel stressed!' – but keep reassuring it that you're trying something different this time and ask it to gently step back and give the other parts a chance.

The more you practise, and the more the new parts are given the opportunity to help, the easier it'll become. The stressed part will then be able to build up trust in these other parts, realise that it doesn't have to carry the whole burden alone, and slowly relinquish its hold on the controls, thereby letting your levels of stress reduce.

Summary

■ Every part has positive intent.

■ Always thank the part for the work that it's doing;
it will feel that its role is helping you, so telling it off
won't help.

■ Notice the age of your part so you know how best to
communicate with it.

■ Remember your stressed part is just a part of you, not
all of you, so you can recruit other parts to help it.

■ See which other parts are best suited to help.

■ Remember, the more you practise the easier and
quicker it'll be to soothe your stressed parts.

8 How to sleep when you're stressed

We've heard it so many times before from so many people: 'If you get more sleep, better quality sleep, deeper sleep, then you'll feel better in all aspects of your life. With more sleep you won't feel so stressed, you'll be more balanced and calmer and you'll be better able to cope with whatever life throws at you'. This is all nice in theory but when you're lying in bed awake at 3 a.m., with your mind buzzing and sleep seeming a million miles away, it doesn't matter that you *know* sleep is good for you; what matters is if you can actually get any.

Stress is a huge factor in fuelling sleep deprivation, and it's a vicious cycle: you know that sleep will help you feel better, but you can't get to sleep so you get stressed about needing sleep, and that stress keeps you awake. Then, even the idea of going to bed knowing you need to sleep and you've only got a certain number of hours to do so, starts stressing you out, so you employ all sorts of tactics to try and tire yourself out – watching TV until it's very late, having a glass of wine. . . then another. And yet sleep still eludes you, *and* you're falling into unhealthy habits. Being awake in the middle of the night, when all you want is to be asleep, adds another mountain of stress to any already overstressed brain.

Deactivate your mind

Falling asleep when you're in a heightened state of arousal is almost impossible. The reason for the fight or flight response – which is activated when you're stressed – is to save you from imminent danger. What good would it be if you were asleep when you were in danger? When you're stressed, your body believes there's some kind of threat and therefore it feels that you need to stay awake and be alert. Hence, sleep doesn't come. The key is to calm down your body and mind and deactivate the stress response, so your body and mind feel safe, enabling you to go to sleep.

Exercise 8.1
Calm your body

- As with every exercise in this the book, the first thing you need to concentrate on is your breathing. Make sure you are breathing deeply into your stomach and try to empty your mind of all your thoughts.

- Breathe deeply into your abdomen just as you learnt in Exercise 3.2.

- Once your breathing is deep and even, the goal is to relax every aspect of your body, inch by inch.

- Start with your toes. Wriggle your toes gently, then imagine every aspect of them – every bone, every joint, every ligament, every vein – relaxing.

- Move slowly up your feet, again imagine every tiny bone (there are twenty-six of them and over a hundred ligaments, tendons and muscles) relaxing.

■ Move up to your ankles – again imagine every part of them relaxing.

■ Following this pattern, very slowly travel all the way up your body, imagining each part of it one by one, each and every aspect of your body, relaxing and falling into a deep, safe sleep.

■ When you finally get to your head (if you haven't fallen asleep already), then imagine the physical make up of your brain relaxing. Imagine the neurons slowing down and taking some time out from their constant firing. Imagine the lights going out, just like when you turn off the bedroom light. Imagine it's all dark and cosy and safe in there, and imagine your brain slowly going to sleep.

If you notice your mind wandering as you do this, then bring your attention back to your breath; once your mind has calmed down, then quickly remind yourself of all the bits you've relaxed so far then slowly continue up your body. As always, this exercise gets more effective the more often you do it. You might find your first attempt very frustrating, as your mind can constantly interfere, but try not to be judgemental of yourself and persevere.

TOP TIP
If it helps, imagine your body is in your safe place (Chapter 6) before you start relaxing it to ensure that you feel as safe as possible. This will help you relax.

Sleep apps

There are lots of sleep-aid apps available that can help soothe and slow a whizzing mind. Try out a couple and see what resonates the most with you. Before you choose one, spend a bit of time thinking about what creates the perfect scenario for you to go to sleep. It might be that a certain tone of voice relaxes you, yet another might stimulate you; some accents might grate on your nerves, while others sooth you. The sound of water might be calming to one person but to another it just reminds them of being afraid. Everyone will have different things that help them feel safe. Find what yours is, then see if you can find an audio example of it that you can listen to once you're in bed. Practise your deep breathing as you're listening to your chosen sound; you can also combine the auditory relaxation with the body relaxation technique from Exercise 8.1 (p.113).

Pamela (41) grew up as an expat in the Philippines. She had a very destructive family, and her resounding childhood memory is of her parents' arguing and physically fighting, which was often her life soundtrack after she went to bed. The only time she felt truly safe was when she was with the Filipino nanny who epitomised maternal love. And the only time she easily fell into a deep sleep was when the nanny was with her, quietly chatting on the phone in Filipino, a language Pamela didn't understand. The gentle undulations of the language lulled Pamela to sleep; the fact that she couldn't understand what was being said added to the soporific effect as her mind was able to let the chatter drift into background noise. When she came to me as an adult, Pamela was very stressed and lack of sleep was one of her symptoms. After discovering tools to help her feel safe at night, she found an audio book that was in Filipino and tried playing it once she was in bed. The sounds soothed her mind and transformed her sleeping, which in turn helped her better manage the stress of her daily life.

Routine is essential

Our bodies and minds love routine and respond to it very well. Just as with young children, having a consistent bedtime routine is hugely beneficial to getting a good night's sleep. If you go to bed at the same time every day, then your body will know that it's time to start winding down and it will naturally start getting ready to rest. Of course, for a lot of people it's not possible to be totally rigid on what time you go to bed, but where possible make a regular bedtime a priority. Also stick to the same bedtime routine everyday – washing your face, brushing your teeth, having a bath – whatever it is that you do, be consistent (and this you *can* stick to whatever time you go to bed). Again, this repetitive behaviour will send signals to your brain that you're getting ready to go to sleep. Consciously practise your deep breathing as you go through your routine to help your body get into a calm state before bed.

Harmonise your room

Leave your phone, tablet, and all electronic devices that you associate with feeling stressed, out of your room. Just knowing that they are next to you can set your mind racing and stop you going to sleep. Glancing at the time in the middle of the night and seeing a message from your boss/your former partner can send your mind into a spin, activating your stress levels and preventing any more sleep. Simply take this option out of the equation by not having the device anywhere near you. If you do need to do any late-night, last-minute work, keep this out of the bedroom. Make sure you have a firm boundary in place that your bedroom is only used for sleeping and relaxing. Anything that might cause stress, activate you and wake you up needs to be taken into another room. Again, this will help your body and mind associate your bedroom with sleep, and it will be more inclined to slip into restful mode when it's in there.

Switch up your energy

If you've been lying there trying to go to sleep for over thirty minutes with no success, then instead of winding yourself up by getting angry and frustrated, which will just wake you up further, switch up what you're doing. Turn on a dim light and read a book until you feel your eyes going heavy and you begin to feel drowsy; or switch from doing a meditation to using an audio sleep aid; or go and get a glass of water (without turning on any bright lights), practise some breathing, then come back to the bedroom and try again.

Empty your head

If your mind is buzzing, then jot down a few notes on a pad next to your bed. Once they're on paper you can be reassured you won't forget anything thus allowing the racing thoughts to leave your mind until the morning. Then focus all your attention on your breath and try and clear your mind so you can more easily fall asleep.

Summary

- Deactivate your mind using your breath.

- Focus on relaxing your whole body inch by inch.

- Use your safe space to let your body know it's okay to go to sleep.

- Try a sleep app that is tailored to your own history of feeling safe when asleep.

- Stick to a routine.

- Keep your room a sleep-only space – no work allowed!

- Take notes of your thoughts so they're on paper and can leave your head.

- If none of the above have worked, try to stay as calm as possible and attempt a different tactic.

Final thoughts

Our minds and bodies are so intricately connected that the best way to move forwards with any issue shrouded in stress is to tune into both of them. Be open and curious about your reactions to anything (both positive and negative) – your mind and body are trying to tell you something, so give yourself the chance to listen to what they are trying to say. Ultimately, our beings are striving for optimum health, so if something is causing you distress then, instead of sweeping it under the carpet and ignoring it, go towards it and explore it so you can find a way to deal with it, heal and move forwards.

Combine techniques

Once you've had a go at trying all the techniques in this book on their own, start combining them. For example, if you have identified your core beliefs, then you can start to be curious about which part of you is holding that belief. Always use the deep breathing techniques, as this will physically help you reduce stress in every scenario. Once you know a core belief, then try being in the now with it: 'I'm going to be late, which means I'm disrespectful; but in this moment, right now, I am here in this car and I am okay. Therefore, I can cope with this and I'll deal with my mother's disappointment as and when it happens, *if* it happens.'

Expand these exercises to all aspects of your life

Now that you have all the tools to really connect to yourself, make the most of them and use them in every aspect of your life, not just when you're feeling stressed. For example, if you're experiencing extreme happiness or contentment, then allow it to flood your whole being and enjoy the feeling as it radiates from every aspect of your being. Notice and enjoy the parts of yourself that come into play when you're really happy; enjoy the contentment and connection you feel when you're happy and living in the NOW. Also notice and enjoy the increased energy you feel when you're not wasting it all on being stressed!

Resources

- Chödrön, P., *Start Where You Are* (Element, 2016)

- Hanson, R., *Hardwiring Happiness* (Rider, 2014)

- van der Kolk, B., *The Body Keeps the Score: Mind, Brain and Body in the Transformation of Trauma* (Allen Lane, 2015)

- McKay, M., Wood J. C. & Brantley J., *The Dialectical Behavior Therapy Skills Workbook* (New Harbinger Publications, 2019)

- Schwartz, R. C. & Sweezy M., *Internal Family Systems Therapy* (The Guilford Press, 2019)

- Tolle, E., *The Power of Now* (Yellow Kite, 2020)

Notes